Essential Oils
70 Recipes Every Essential Oil Beginner Should Try

Table of content

Introduction

You're familiar with essential oils. You know they can be used in a variety of natural remedies, a variety of natural cleaners, and a variety of natural air cleansers, but you may not know how to make this happen.

Of course, you want to make blends that smell great, but when it comes to the hundreds of essential oils that are out there in the world, you may not know where to start. There are so many spices, mints, and flowers, so many trees, plants, and even chocolates that they have turned into essential oils.

When it comes to which one you are going to use with another, it can be hard to know where to start.

"I don't want to waste oils in a blend that doesn't turn out."

"I don't want to spend money to get an oil if I don't know what to blend it with."

"I don't know which oils to blend in my diffuser."

Of course, if you know anything about essential oils, you know it really doesn't matter what you do, as long as you are happy with the results, but when it comes to putting together blends you know are going to turn out, it can be a whole new story.

And that's where this book comes in. In it, I am going to show you just what you need to do to make the blends of your dreams. I am going to show you how to use oils to fill your house with rich, warm scents while you use entirely natural products, and I am going to show you how to use the simple oils you have on hand already to make that happen.

It's incredible how many blends you can create with basic oils that are easy to find nearly everywhere, and it's incredibly how rich and wonderful you can make your home smell with just the right kinds of oils.

With this book, nothing is going to stop you. Mix and match the oils, mix and match the recipes, and mix and match your creativity to get the best results, and fall in love with the blends you create. There's no end to the ways you can express yourself through your oils, and when it comes to the results you experience, you will be hooked from the very first blend.

So go ahead, indulge a little.

Chapter 1 – Beginner Blends

Basic Beauty

What you will need:

10 drops rose oil

8 drops roman chamomile

3 drops rosewood

Directions:

Combine your oils in a dark bottle if you are going to store them over a longer period of time, or mix directly in your diffuser.

Plug into your diffuser and let the rich scent fill the room, or your entire house! There's no limit to the amount of diffusers you can have, so run wild.

If you would like to apply directly to your skin, mix with 1 teaspoon of a carrier oil of your choice before applying. Spread evenly over your forehead or your jawline, or massage into your shoulders.

Fashion Sense

What you will need:

10 drops lavender oil

8 drops lilac oil

5 drops sunflower essential oil

Directions:

Combine your oils in a dark bottle if you are going to store them over a longer period of time, or mix directly in your diffuser.

Plug into your diffuser and let the rich scent fill the room, or your entire house! There's no limit to the amount of diffusers you can have, so run wild.

If you would like to apply directly to your skin, mix with 1 teaspoon of a carrier oil of your choice before applying. Spread evenly over your forehead or your jawline, or massage into your shoulders.

Sensation Station

What you will need:

10 drops peppermint oil

6 drops lavender oil

5 drops vetiver oil

Directions:

Combine your oils in a dark bottle if you are going to store them over a longer period of time, or mix directly in your diffuser.

Plug into your diffuser and let the rich scent fill the room, or your entire house! There's no limit to the amount of diffusers you can have, so run wild.

If you would like to apply directly to your skin, mix with 1 teaspoon of a carrier oil of your choice before applying. Spread evenly over your forehead or your jawline, or massage into your shoulders.

Guilt-free Goodness

What you will need:

10 drops sweet orange oil

8 drops lemon

8 drops lemongrass

Directions:

Combine your oils in a dark bottle if you are going to store them over a longer period of time, or mix directly in your diffuser.

Plug into your diffuser and let the rich scent fill the room, or your entire house! There's no limit to the amount of diffusers you can have, so run wild.

If you would like to apply directly to your skin, mix with 1 teaspoon of a carrier oil of your choice before applying. Spread evenly over your forehead or your jawline, or massage into your shoulders.

The Happy Blend

What you will need:

10 drops vetiver oil

8 drops ylang ylang

7 drops geranium oil

Directions:

Combine your oils in a dark bottle if you are going to store them over a longer period of time, or mix directly in your diffuser.

Plug into your diffuser and let the rich scent fill the room, or your entire house! There's no limit to the amount of diffusers you can have, so run wild.

If you would like to apply directly to your skin, mix with 1 teaspoon of a carrier oil of your choice before applying. Spread evenly over your forehead or your jawline, or massage into your shoulders.

Undercover Agent

What you will need:

10 drops chamomile

8 drops bergamot oil

8 drops helichrysum

Directions:

Combine your oils in a dark bottle if you are going to store them over a longer period of time, or mix directly in your diffuser.

Plug into your diffuser and let the rich scent fill the room, or your entire house! There's no limit to the amount of diffusers you can have, so run wild.

If you would like to apply directly to your skin, mix with 1 teaspoon of a carrier oil of your choice before applying. Spread evenly over your forehead or your jawline, or massage into your shoulders.

The Answer to Everything

What you will need:

10 drops frankincense

8 drops rosemary oil

8 drops sandalwood

Directions:

Combine your oils in a dark bottle if you are going to store them over a longer period of time, or mix directly in your diffuser.

Plug into your diffuser and let the rich scent fill the room, or your entire house! There's no limit to the amount of diffusers you can have, so run wild.

If you would like to apply directly to your skin, mix with 1 teaspoon of a carrier oil of your choice before applying. Spread evenly over your forehead or your jawline, or massage into your shoulders.

Magic Mix

What you will need:

10 drops basil oil

8 drops cardamom oil

8 drops geranium oil

Directions:

Combine your oils in a dark bottle if you are going to store them over a longer period of time, or mix directly in your diffuser.

Plug into your diffuser and let the rich scent fill the room, or your entire house! There's no limit to the amount of diffusers you can have, so run wild.

If you would like to apply directly to your skin, mix with 1 teaspoon of a carrier oil of your choice before applying. Spread evenly over your forehead or your jawline, or massage into your shoulders.

Chapter 2 – Diffuser Blends

Peppermint Paradise

What you will need:

12 drops peppermint

10 drops spearmint

8 drops vanilla

Directions:

Combine your oils in a dark bottle if you are going to store them over a longer period of time, or mix directly in your diffuser.

Plug in your diffuser and let the aroma fill the air as the rich scent permeates through your home. Keep in one room of your house or place in several rooms of the house for a perfectly peaceful atmosphere in your entire home!

Fresh Air

What you will need:

10 drops pine

10 drops winter green oil

10 drops spruce

Directions:

Combine your oils in a dark bottle if you are going to store them over a longer period of time, or mix directly in your diffuser.

Plug in your diffuser and let the aroma fill the air as the rich scent permeates through your home. Keep in one room of your house or place in several rooms of the house for a perfectly peaceful atmosphere in your entire home!

Sunshine

What you will need:

10 drops hibiscus oil

8 drops jasmine oil

8 drops star anise oil

Directions:

Combine your oils in a dark bottle if you are going to store them over a longer period of time, or mix directly in your diffuser.

Plug in your diffuser and let the aroma fill the air as the rich scent permeates through your home. Keep in one room of your house or place in several rooms of the house for a perfectly peaceful atmosphere in your entire home!

Holiday Bash

What you will need:

10 drops cinnamon

10 drops nutmeg

8 drops vanilla

Directions:

Combine your oils in a dark bottle if you are going to store them over a longer period of time, or mix directly in your diffuser.

Plug in your diffuser and let the aroma fill the air as the rich scent permeates through your home. Keep in one room of your house or place in several rooms of the house for a perfectly peaceful atmosphere in your entire home!

Christmas Carols

What you will need:

10 drops peppermint oil

10 drops cacao essential oi

8 drops vanilla essential oil

Directions:

Combine your oils in a dark bottle if you are going to store them over a longer period of time, or mix directly in your diffuser.

Plug in your diffuser and let the aroma fill the air as the rich scent permeates through your home. Keep in one room of your house or place in several rooms of the house for a perfectly peaceful atmosphere in your entire home!

Holly Jolly Christmas

What you will need:

10 drops peppermint

8 drops cinnamon

8 drops spruce oil

Directions:

Combine your oils in a dark bottle if you are going to store them over a longer period of time, or mix directly in your diffuser.

Plug in your diffuser and let the aroma fill the air as the rich scent permeates through your home. Keep in one room of your house or place in several rooms of the house for a perfectly peaceful atmosphere in your entire home!

Yuletide Joy

What you will need:

10 drops peppermint

9 drops pine

9 drops fir needle

Directions:

Combine your oils in a dark bottle if you are going to store them over a longer period of time, or mix directly in your diffuser.

Plug in your diffuser and let the aroma fill the air as the rich scent permeates through your home. Keep in one room of your house or place in several rooms of the house for a perfectly peaceful atmosphere in your entire home!

Crackling Fire

What you will need:

20 drops sandalwood

10 drops spruce

10 drops fir needle

Directions:

Combine your oils in a dark bottle if you are going to store them over a longer period of time, or mix directly in your diffuser.

Plug in your diffuser and let the aroma fill the air as the rich scent permeates through your home. Keep in one room of your house or place in several rooms of the house for a perfectly peaceful atmosphere in your entire home!

Chapter 3 – Wellness Blends

Headache Healer

What you will need:

10 drops peppermint

8 drops lavender

8 drops lemon oil

Directions:

Combine your oils in a dark bottle if you are going to store them over a longer period of time, or mix directly in your diffuser.

Plug into your diffuser and let the rich scent fill the room, or your entire house! There's no limit to the amount of diffusers you can have, so run wild.

If you would like to apply directly to your skin, mix with 1 teaspoon of a carrier oil of your choice before applying. Spread evenly over your forehead or your jawline, or massage into your shoulders.

Aches and Pains Banisher

What you will need:

10 drops myrrh

8 drops frankincense

8 drops goldenseal

Directions:

Combine your oils in a dark bottle if you are going to store them over a longer period of time, or mix directly in your diffuser.

Plug into your diffuser and let the rich scent fill the room, or your entire house! There's no limit to the amount of diffusers you can have, so run wild.

If you would like to apply directly to your skin, mix with 1 teaspoon of a carrier oil of your choice before applying. Spread evenly over your forehead or your jawline, or massage into your shoulders.

Feel Good Blend

What you will need:

10 drops eucalyptus

12 drops lavender

8 drops spearmint

Directions:

Combine your oils in a dark bottle if you are going to store them over a longer period of time, or mix directly in your diffuser.

Plug into your diffuser and let the rich scent fill the room, or your entire house! There's no limit to the amount of diffusers you can have, so run wild.

If you would like to apply directly to your skin, mix with 1 teaspoon of a carrier oil of your choice before applying. Spread evenly over your forehead or your jawline, or massage into your shoulders.

Clear Mind and Soul

What you will need:

10 drops mint

8 drops vetiver

8 drops helichrysum

Directions:

Combine your oils in a dark bottle if you are going to store them over a longer period of time, or mix directly in your diffuser.

Plug into your diffuser and let the rich scent fill the room, or your entire house! There's no limit to the amount of diffusers you can have, so run wild.

If you would like to apply directly to your skin, mix with 1 teaspoon of a carrier oil of your choice before applying. Spread evenly over your forehead or your jawline, or massage into your shoulders.

Health and Happiness

What you will need:

10 drops grapefruit

8 drops orange

8 drops sweet orange

Directions:

Combine your oils in a dark bottle if you are going to store them over a longer period of time, or mix directly in your diffuser.

Plug into your diffuser and let the rich scent fill the room, or your entire house! There's no limit to the amount of diffusers you can have, so run wild.

If you would like to apply directly to your skin, mix with 1 teaspoon of a carrier oil of your choice before applying. Spread evenly over your forehead or your jawline, or massage into your shoulders.

Thin and Trim

What you will need:

10 drops ginger

8 drops cinnamon

8 drops vanilla

8 drops sweet orange

Directions:

Combine your oils in a dark bottle if you are going to store them over a longer period of time, or mix directly in your diffuser.

Plug into your diffuser and let the rich scent fill the room, or your entire house! There's no limit to the amount of diffusers you can have, so run wild.

If you would like to apply directly to your skin, mix with 1 teaspoon of a carrier oil of your choice before applying. Spread evenly over your forehead or your jawline, or massage into your shoulders.

Cold Basher Blast

What you will need:

10 drops orange

10 drops sweet orange

8 drops blood orange oil

Directions:

Combine your oils in a dark bottle if you are going to store them over a longer period of time, or mix directly in your diffuser.

Plug into your diffuser and let the rich scent fill the room, or your entire house! There's no limit to the amount of diffusers you can have, so run wild.

If you would like to apply directly to your skin, mix with 1 teaspoon of a carrier oil of your choice before applying. Spread evenly over your forehead or your jawline, or massage into your shoulders.

Chapter 4 – Bath and Body Blends

Clear Skin

What you will need:

10 drops myrrh oil

8 drops tea tree oil

8 drops vetiver

Directions:

Combine your oils in a dark bottle if you are going to store them over a longer period of time, or mix directly in your diffuser.

Plug into your diffuser and let the rich scent fill the room, or your entire house! There's no limit to the amount of diffusers you can have, so run wild.

If you would like to apply directly to your skin, mix with 1 teaspoon of a carrier oil of your choice before applying. Spread evenly over your forehead or your jawline, or massage into your shoulders.

High Hair

What you will need:

8 drops tea tree oil

8 drops marjoram

8 drops jasmine

Directions:

Combine your oils in a dark bottle if you are going to store them over a longer period of time, or mix directly in your diffuser.

Plug into your diffuser and let the rich scent fill the room, or your entire house! There's no limit to the amount of diffusers you can have, so run wild.

If you would like to apply directly to your skin, mix with 1 teaspoon of a carrier oil of your choice before applying. Spread evenly over your forehead or your jawline, or massage into your shoulders.

Wrinkle Washout

What you will need:

10 drops myrrh oil

9 drops lemon

8 drops tea tree oil

Directions:

Combine your oils in a dark bottle if you are going to store them over a longer period of time, or mix directly in your diffuser.

Plug into your diffuser and let the rich scent fill the room, or your entire house! There's no limit to the amount of diffusers you can have, so run wild.

If you would like to apply directly to your skin, mix with 1 teaspoon of a carrier oil of your choice before applying. Spread evenly over your forehead or your jawline, or massage into your shoulders.

Youthfulness

What you will need:

10 drops ylang ylang

8 drops cardamom

8 drops helichrysum

Directions:

Combine your oils in a dark bottle if you are going to store them over a longer period of time, or mix directly in your diffuser.

Plug into your diffuser and let the rich scent fill the room, or your entire house! There's no limit to the amount of diffusers you can have, so run wild.

If you would like to apply directly to your skin, mix with 1 teaspoon of a carrier oil of your choice before applying. Spread evenly over your forehead or your jawline, or massage into your shoulders.

Blemish Remover Blend

What you will need:

10 drops eucalyptus oil

8 drops myrrh oil

8 drops grapefruit oil

Directions:

Combine your oils in a dark bottle if you are going to store them over a longer period of time, or mix directly in your diffuser.

Plug into your diffuser and let the rich scent fill the room, or your entire house! There's no limit to the amount of diffusers you can have, so run wild.

If you would like to apply directly to your skin, mix with 1 teaspoon of a carrier oil of your choice before applying. Spread evenly over your forehead or your jawline, or massage into your shoulders.

Just You

What you will need:

10 drops geranium

10 drops bergamot

9 drops cedar

Directions:

Combine your oils in a dark bottle if you are going to store them over a longer period of time, or mix directly in your diffuser.

Plug into your diffuser and let the rich scent fill the room, or your entire house! There's no limit to the amount of diffusers you can have, so run wild.

If you would like to apply directly to your skin, mix with 1 teaspoon of a carrier oil of your choice before applying. Spread evenly over your forehead or your jawline, or massage into your shoulders.

Namaste

What you will need:

10 drops hibiscus

10 drops jasmine

10 drops lemon

10 drops lavender

Directions:

Combine your oils in a dark bottle if you are going to store them over a longer period of time, or mix directly in your diffuser.

Plug into your diffuser and let the rich scent fill the room, or your entire house! There's no limit to the amount of diffusers you can have, so run wild.

If you would like to apply directly to your skin, mix with 1 teaspoon of a carrier oil of your choice before applying. Spread evenly over your forehead or your jawline, or massage into your shoulders.

Glorious Greatness

What you will need:

8 drops goldenseal

8 drops vanilla

8 drops neroli

Directions:

Combine your oils in a dark bottle if you are going to store them over a longer period of time, or mix directly in your diffuser.

Plug into your diffuser and let the rich scent fill the room, or your entire house! There's no limit to the amount of diffusers you can have, so run wild.

If you would like to apply directly to your skin, mix with 1 teaspoon of a carrier oil of your choice before applying. Spread evenly over your forehead or your jawline, or massage into your shoulders.

Chapter 5 – Best of the Rest

King's Blend

What you will need:

10 drops rosewood

10 drops cedarwood

10 drops sandalwood

Directions:

Combine your oils in a dark bottle if you are going to store them over a longer period of time, or mix directly in your diffuser.

Plug into your diffuser and let the rich scent fill the room, or your entire house! There's no limit to the amount of diffusers you can have, so run wild.

If you would like to apply directly to your skin, mix with 1 teaspoon of a carrier oil of your choice before applying. Spread evenly over your forehead or your jawline, or massage into your shoulders.

For the Family

What you will need:

10 drops ginger

10 drops frankincense

8 drops roman chamomile

Directions:

Combine your oils in a dark bottle if you are going to store them over a longer period of time, or mix directly in your diffuser.

Plug into your diffuser and let the rich scent fill the room, or your entire house! There's no limit to the amount of diffusers you can have, so run wild.

If you would like to apply directly to your skin, mix with 1 teaspoon of a carrier oil of your choice before applying. Spread evenly over your forehead or your jawline, or massage into your shoulders.

Fantasy

What you will need:

10 drops vetiver oil

9 drops neroli

4 drops basil

Directions:

Combine your oils in a dark bottle if you are going to store them over a longer period of time, or mix directly in your diffuser.

Plug into your diffuser and let the rich scent fill the room, or your entire house! There's no limit to the amount of diffusers you can have, so run wild.

If you would like to apply directly to your skin, mix with 1 teaspoon of a carrier oil of your choice before applying. Spread evenly over your forehead or your jawline, or massage into your shoulders.

Total Healing

What you will need:

9 drops tea tree oil

8 drops ginger oil

8 drops garlic oil

Directions:

Combine your oils in a dark bottle if you are going to store them over a longer period of time, or mix directly in your diffuser.

Plug into your diffuser and let the rich scent fill the room, or your entire house! There's no limit to the amount of diffusers you can have, so run wild.

If you would like to apply directly to your skin, mix with 1 teaspoon of a carrier oil of your choice before applying. Spread evenly over your forehead or your jawline, or massage into your shoulders.

What She Said

What you will need:

10 drops pine needle

8 drops spruce

8 drops lilac

3 drops rose

Directions:

Combine your oils in a dark bottle if you are going to store them over a longer period of time, or mix directly in your diffuser.

Plug into your diffuser and let the rich scent fill the room, or your entire house! There's no limit to the amount of diffusers you can have, so run wild.

If you would like to apply directly to your skin, mix with 1 teaspoon of a carrier oil of your choice before applying. Spread evenly over your forehead or your jawline, or massage into your shoulders.

Jump for Joy

What you will need:

10 drops star anise

9 drops jasmine

8 drops grapefruit

Directions:

Combine your oils in a dark bottle if you are going to store them over a longer period of time, or mix directly in your diffuser.

Plug into your diffuser and let the rich scent fill the room, or your entire house! There's no limit to the amount of diffusers you can have, so run wild.

If you would like to apply directly to your skin, mix with 1 teaspoon of a carrier oil of your choice before applying. Spread evenly over your forehead or your jawline, or massage into your shoulders.

Over and Under

What you will need:

10 drops lemon

9 drops geranium

9 drops ylang ylang

Directions:

Combine your oils in a dark bottle if you are going to store them over a longer period of time, or mix directly in your diffuser.

Plug into your diffuser and let the rich scent fill the room, or your entire house! There's no limit to the amount of diffusers you can have, so run wild.

If you would like to apply directly to your skin, mix with 1 teaspoon of a carrier oil of your choice before applying. Spread evenly over your forehead or your jawline, or massage into your shoulders.

Just in Time

What you will need:

10 drops parsley

9 drops basil

8 drops cinnamon

8 drops vanilla

Directions:

Combine your oils in a dark bottle if you are going to store them over a longer period of time, or mix directly in your diffuser.

Plug into your diffuser and let the rich scent fill the room, or your entire house! There's no limit to the amount of diffusers you can have, so run wild.

If you would like to apply directly to your skin, mix with 1 teaspoon of a carrier oil of your choice before applying. Spread evenly over your forehead or your jawline, or massage into your shoulders.

Chapter 6 – Essential Oil for Health

The Good Day Blend

What you will need:

8 drops lavender oil

3 drops tea tree oil

8 drops roman chamomile oil

Directions:

Place 8-12 drops in your diffuser with some water and plug in. Let the aroma fill the air and breathe in the wellness and healing.

If you would like to apply directly to your skin, make sure you mix with a carrier oil such as fractionated coconut oil, or sweet almond oil. Mix 3 drops essentials with 6 drops carrier oil, and spread across your forehead.

Mix 1 drop per eight ounces tea for a warming healing drink... only use internally with great caution!

Another great way to indulge in these oils is with 10 drops or so in your bath water. Soak up the bliss and enjoy!

Serenity Bliss

What you will need:

10 drops ylang ylang essential oil

8 drops roman chamomile oil

5 drops lavender oil

Directions:

Place 8-12 drops in your diffuser with some water and plug in. Let the aroma fill the air and breathe in the wellness and healing.

If you would like to apply directly to your skin, make sure you mix with a carrier oil such as fractionated coconut oil, or sweet almond oil. Mix 3 drops essentials with 6 drops carrier oil, and spread across your forehead.

Mix 1 drop per eight ounces tea for a warming healing drink... only use internally with great caution!

Another great way to indulge in these oils is with 10 drops or so in your bath water. Soak up the bliss and enjoy!

Happy Health

What you will need:

10 drops frankincense essential oil

8 drops rose essential oil

8 drops ylang ylang oil

5 drops lavender oil

Directions:

Place 8-12 drops in your diffuser with some water and plug in. Let the aroma fill the air and breathe in the wellness and healing.

If you would like to apply directly to your skin, make sure you mix with a carrier oil such as fractionated coconut oil, or sweet almond oil. Mix 3 drops essentials with 6 drops carrier oil, and spread across your forehead.

Mix 1 drop per eight ounces tea for a warming healing drink... only use internally with great caution!

Another great way to indulge in these oils is with 10 drops or so in your bath water. Soak up the bliss and enjoy!

Peach and Clarity

What you will need:

10 drops rose essential oil

8 drops bergamot essential oil

8 drops orange essential oil

Directions:

Place 8-12 drops in your diffuser with some water and plug in. Let the aroma fill the air and breathe in the wellness and healing.

If you would like to apply directly to your skin, make sure you mix with a carrier oil such as fractionated coconut oil, or sweet almond oil. Mix 3 drops essentials with 6 drops carrier oil, and spread across your forehead.

Mix 1 drop per eight ounces tea for a warming healing drink... only use internally with great caution!

Another great way to indulge in these oils is with 10 drops or so in your bath water. Soak up the bliss and enjoy!

Hopeful Happiness

What you will need:

10 drops basil essential oil

10 drops bergamot essential oil

8 drops rose essential oil

Directions:

Place 8-12 drops in your diffuser with some water and plug in. Let the aroma fill the air and breathe in the wellness and healing.

If you would like to apply directly to your skin, make sure you mix with a carrier oil such as fractionated coconut oil, or sweet almond oil. Mix 3 drops essentials with 6 drops carrier oil, and spread across your forehead.

Mix 1 drop per eight ounces tea for a warming healing drink... only use internally with great caution!

Another great way to indulge in these oils is with 10 drops or so in your bath water. Soak up the bliss and enjoy!

Chapter 7 – Weight and Wellness

Happy Scale

What you will need:

10 drops grapefruit essential oil

10 drops rosemary essential oil

8 drops lemon essential oil

Directions:

Place 8-12 drops in your diffuser with some water and plug in. Let the aroma fill the air and breathe in the wellness and healing.

If you would like to apply directly to your skin, make sure you mix with a carrier oil such as fractionated coconut oil, or sweet almond oil. Mix 3 drops essentials with 6 drops carrier oil, and spread across your forehead.

Mix 1 drop per eight ounces tea for a warming healing drink... only use internally with great caution!

Another great way to indulge in these oils is with 10 drops or so in your bath water. Soak up the bliss and enjoy!

Good Tummy Blend

What you will need:

10 drops peppermint essential oil

8 drops ginger essential oil

5 drops spearmint essential oil

Directions:

Place 8-12 drops in your diffuser with some water and plug in. Let the aroma fill the air and breathe in the wellness and healing.

If you would like to apply directly to your skin, make sure you mix with a carrier oil such as fractionated coconut oil, or sweet almond oil. Mix 3 drops essentials with 6 drops carrier oil, and spread across your forehead.

Mix 1 drop per eight ounces tea for a warming healing drink... only use internally with great caution!

Another great way to indulge in these oils is with 10 drops or so in your bath water. Soak up the bliss and enjoy!

Skinny Jean

What you will need:

10 drops rosewood essential oil

10 drops rose essential oil

8 drops rosemary essential oil

Directions:

Place 8-12 drops in your diffuser with some water and plug in. Let the aroma fill the air and breathe in the wellness and healing.

If you would like to apply directly to your skin, make sure you mix with a carrier oil such as fractionated coconut oil, or sweet almond oil. Mix 3 drops essentials with 6 drops carrier oil, and spread across your forehead.

Mix 1 drop per eight ounces tea for a warming healing drink... only use internally with great caution!

Another great way to indulge in these oils is with 10 drops or so in your bath water. Soak up the bliss and enjoy!

Eat What You Want

What you will need:

10 drops cypress essential oil

10 drops ginger essential oil

8 drops lemon essential oil

Directions:

Place 8-12 drops in your diffuser with some water and plug in. Let the aroma fill the air and breathe in the wellness and healing.

If you would like to apply directly to your skin, make sure you mix with a carrier oil such as fractionated coconut oil, or sweet almond oil. Mix 3 drops essentials with 6 drops carrier oil, and spread across your forehead.

Mix 1 drop per eight ounces tea for a warming healing drink... only use internally with great caution!

Another great way to indulge in these oils is with 10 drops or so in your bath water. Soak up the bliss and enjoy!

The Luscious Curves

What you will need:

10 drops lemon essential oil

10 drops grapefruit essential oil

8 drops orange essential oil

8 drops blood orange essential oil

Directions:

Place 8-12 drops in your diffuser with some water and plug in. Let the aroma fill the air and breathe in the wellness and healing.

If you would like to apply directly to your skin, make sure you mix with a carrier oil such as fractionated coconut oil, or sweet almond oil. Mix 3 drops essentials with 6 drops carrier oil, and spread across your forehead.

Mix 1 drop per eight ounces tea for a warming healing drink... only use internally with great caution!

Another great way to indulge in these oils is with 10 drops or so in your bath water. Soak up the bliss and enjoy!

Chapter 8 – Beauty Care

The Young Goddess

What you will need:

10 drops cypress essential oil

10 drops myrrh essential oil

8 drops tea tree essential oil

8 drops geranium essential oil

Directions:

Place 8-12 drops in your diffuser with some water and plug in. Let the aroma fill the air and breathe in the wellness and healing.

If you would like to apply directly to your skin, make sure you mix with a carrier oil such as fractionated coconut oil, or sweet almond oil. Mix 3 drops essentials with 6 drops carrier oil, and spread across your forehead, and on your cheeks... be careful under your eyes.

Mix 1 drop per eight ounces tea for a warming healing drink... only use internally with great caution!

Another great way to indulge in these oils is with 10 drops or so in your bath water. Soak up the bliss and enjoy!

Clear Skin Wonder

What you will need:

10 drops tea tree oil

10 drops myrrh oil

8 drops goldenseal essential oil

Directions:

Place 8-12 drops in your diffuser with some water and plug in. Let the aroma fill the air and breathe in the wellness and healing.

If you would like to apply directly to your skin, make sure you mix with a carrier oil such as fractionated coconut oil, or sweet almond oil. Mix 3 drops essentials with 6 drops carrier oil, and spread across your forehead or directly on any breakout.

Mix 1 drop per eight ounces tea for a warming healing drink... only use internally with great caution!

Another great way to indulge in these oils is with 10 drops or so in your bath water. Soak up the bliss and enjoy!

Blemish Blaster

What you will need:

10 drops boswellia

8 drops tea tree oil

8 drops sacra oil

8 drops myrrh oil

Directions:

Place 8-12 drops in your diffuser with some water and plug in. Let the aroma fill the air and breathe in the wellness and healing.

If you would like to apply directly to your skin, make sure you mix with a carrier oil such as fractionated coconut oil, or sweet almond oil. Mix 3 drops essentials with 6 drops carrier oil, and spread across your forehead or directly on any breakout.

Mix 1 drop per eight ounces tea for a warming healing drink... only use internally with great caution!

Another great way to indulge in these oils is with 10 drops or so in your bath water. Soak up the bliss and enjoy!

The Youthful Glow

What you will need:

10 drops frankincense

10 drops myrrh essential oil

8 drops geranium essential oil

8 drops goldenseal essential oil

Directions:

Place 8-12 drops in your diffuser with some water and plug in. Let the aroma fill the air and breathe in the wellness and healing.

If you would like to apply directly to your skin, make sure you mix with a carrier oil such as fractionated coconut oil, or sweet almond oil. Mix 3 drops essentials with 6 drops carrier oil, and spread across your forehead.

Mix 1 drop per eight ounces tea for a warming healing drink... only use internally with great caution!

Another great way to indulge in these oils is with 10 drops or so in your bath water. Soak up the bliss and enjoy!

Fair Skinned Maiden

What you will need:

10 drops grapefruit oil

5 drops geranium essential oil

8 drops tea tree oil

3 drops cinnamon essential oil

Directions:

Place 8-12 drops in your diffuser with some water and plug in. Let the aroma fill the air and breathe in the wellness and healing.

If you would like to apply directly to your skin, make sure you mix with a carrier oil such as fractionated coconut oil, or sweet almond oil. Mix 3 drops essentials with 6 drops carrier oil, and spread across your forehead.

Mix 1 drop per eight ounces tea for a warming healing drink... only use internally with great caution!

Another great way to indulge in these oils is with 10 drops or so in your bath water. Soak up the bliss and enjoy!

Chapter 9 – Around the House

Clean Air

What you will need:

10 drops peppermint essential oil

10 drops eucalyptus oil

10 drops pine oil

5 drops winter green oil

Directions:

Place 8-12 drops in your diffuser with some water and plug in. Let the aroma fill the air and breathe in the wellness and healing.

If you would like to apply directly to your skin, make sure you mix with a carrier oil such as fractionated coconut oil, or sweet almond oil. Mix 3 drops essentials with 6 drops carrier oil, and spread across your forehead.

Mix 1 drop per eight ounces tea for a warming healing drink... only use internally with great caution!

Another great way to indulge in these oils is with 10 drops or so in your bath water. Soak up the bliss and enjoy!

Oasis Shelter

What you will need:

10 drops lemon essential oil

5 drops lemongrass essential oil

5 drops peppermint essential oil

Directions:

Place 8-12 drops in your diffuser with some water and plug in. Let the aroma fill the air and breathe in the wellness and healing.

If you would like to apply directly to your skin, make sure you mix with a carrier oil such as fractionated coconut oil, or sweet almond oil. Mix 3 drops essentials with 6 drops carrier oil, and spread across your forehead.

Mix 1 drop per eight ounces tea for a warming healing drink... only use internally with great caution!

Another great way to indulge in these oils is with 10 drops or so in your bath water. Soak up the bliss and enjoy!

Home is Where the Happiness Is

What you will need:

10 drops rose essential oil

10 drops peppermint essential oil

5 drops lavender essential oil

5 drops lilac essential oil

Directions:

Place 8-12 drops in your diffuser with some water and plug in. Let the aroma fill the air and breathe in the wellness and healing.

If you would like to apply directly to your skin, make sure you mix with a carrier oil such as fractionated coconut oil, or sweet almond oil. Mix 3 drops essentials with 6 drops carrier oil, and spread across your forehead.

Mix 1 drop per eight ounces tea for a warming healing drink... only use internally with great caution!

Another great way to indulge in these oils is with 10 drops or so in your bath water. Soak up the bliss and enjoy!

Stress Away

What you will need:

10 drops roman chamomile

10 drops rose oil

10 drops sunflower essential oil

10 drops cinnamon essential oil

Directions:

Place 8-12 drops in your diffuser with some water and plug in. Let the aroma fill the air and breathe in the wellness and healing.

If you would like to apply directly to your skin, make sure you mix with a carrier oil such as fractionated coconut oil, or sweet almond oil. Mix 3 drops essentials with 6 drops carrier oil, and spread across your forehead.

Mix 1 drop per eight ounces tea for a warming healing drink... only use internally with great caution!

Another great way to indulge in these oils is with 10 drops or so in your bath water. Soak up the bliss and enjoy!

Your Retreat

What you will need:

10 drops bergamot essential oil

10 drops patchouli essential oil

5 drops cedarwood

5 drops sandalwood essential oil

Directions:

Place 8-12 drops in your diffuser with some water and plug in. Let the aroma fill the air and breathe in the wellness and healing.

If you would like to apply directly to your skin, make sure you mix with a carrier oil such as fractionated coconut oil, or sweet almond oil. Mix 3 drops essentials with 6 drops carrier oil, and spread across your forehead.

Mix 1 drop per eight ounces tea for a warming healing drink... only use internally with great caution!

Another great way to indulge in these oils is with 10 drops or so in your bath water. Soak up the bliss and enjoy!

Chapter 10 – For the Kids

Goodnight Blend

What you will need:

10 drops lavender essential oil

5 drops lemon essential oil

Directions:

Place 8-12 drops in your diffuser with some water and plug in. Let the aroma fill the air and breathe in the wellness and healing.

If you would like to apply directly to your skin, make sure you mix with a carrier oil such as fractionated coconut oil, or sweet almond oil. Mix 3 drops essentials with 6 drops carrier oil, and spread across your forehead.

Adults need to be very careful when they use essential oils internally, but it is also very important that you do not let your children ingest any. No tea for the little ones!

The School Day Blend

What you will need:

10 drops peppermint essential oil

5 drops cinnamon essential oil

Directions:

Place 8-12 drops in your diffuser with some water and plug in. Let the aroma fill the air and breathe in the wellness and healing.

If you would like to apply directly to your skin, make sure you mix with a carrier oil such as fractionated coconut oil, or sweet almond oil. Mix 3 drops essentials with 6 drops carrier oil, and spread across your forehead.

Adults need to be very careful when they use essential oils internally, but it is also very important that you do not let your children ingest any. No tea for the little ones!

Mama's Favorite Blend

What you will need:

5 drops tea tree essential oil

15 drops eucalyptus essential oil

5 drops lemon essential oil

Directions:

Place 8-12 drops in your diffuser with some water and plug in. Let the aroma fill the air and breathe in the wellness and healing.

If you would like to apply directly to your skin, make sure you mix with a carrier oil such as fractionated coconut oil, or sweet almond oil. Mix 3 drops essentials with 6 drops carrier oil, and spread across your forehead.

Adults need to be very careful when they use essential oils internally, but it is also very important that you do not let your children ingest any. No tea for the little ones!

The Ouchie Fighter

What you will need:

5 drops tea tree essential oil

10 drops frankincense essential oil

5 drops spikenard essential oil

Directions:

Place 8-12 drops in your diffuser with some water and plug in. Let the aroma fill the air and breathe in the wellness and healing.

If you would like to apply directly to your skin, make sure you mix with a carrier oil such as fractionated coconut oil, or sweet almond oil. Mix 3 drops essentials with 6 drops carrier oil, and spread on the injury site.

Adults need to be very careful when they use essential oils internally, but it is also very important that you do not let your children ingest any. No tea for the little ones!

The Sudsy Blend

What you will need:

10 drops lemon essential oil

5 drops orange essential oil

4 drops rose essential oil

5 drops lavender essential oil

Directions:

Place 8-12 drops in your diffuser with some water and plug in. Let the aroma fill the air and breathe in the wellness and healing.

If you would like to apply directly to your skin, make sure you mix with a carrier oil such as fractionated coconut oil, or sweet almond oil. Mix 3 drops essentials with 6 drops carrier oil, and spread across your forehead.

Adults need to be very careful when they use essential oils internally, but it is also very important that you do not let your children ingest any. No tea for the little ones!

Another great way to indulge in these oils is with 10 drops or so in your bath water. Soak up the bliss and enjoy!

Chapter 11 – Everything Else

Cleaning King

What you will need:

10 drops orange essential oil

8 drops lemon essential oil

5 drops peppermint essential oil

Directions:

Place 8-12 drops in your diffuser with some water and plug in. Let the aroma fill the air and breathe in the wellness and healing.

If you would like to apply directly to your skin, make sure you mix with a carrier oil such as fractionated coconut oil, or sweet almond oil. Mix 3 drops essentials with 6 drops carrier oil, and spread across your forehead.

Mix 1 drop per eight ounces tea for a warming healing drink... only use internally with great caution!

Mix 15 drops with your cleaning water, and let the freshness fill the house!

The Immunity Booster

What you will need:

12 drops thieves oil

10 drops valor

8 drops tea tree essential oil

Directions:

Place 8-12 drops in your diffuser with some water and plug in. Let the aroma fill the air and breathe in the wellness and healing.

If you would like to apply directly to your skin, make sure you mix with a carrier oil such as fractionated coconut oil, or sweet almond oil. Mix 3 drops essentials with 6 drops carrier oil, and spread across your forehead.

Mix 1 drop per eight ounces tea for a warming healing drink... only use internally with great caution!

Another great way to indulge in these oils is with 10 drops or so in your bath water. Soak up the bliss and enjoy!

The All in One

What you will need:

10 drops cinnamon essential oil

10 drops orange essential oil

5 drops bergamot essential oil

5 drops thieves oil

Directions:

Place 8-12 drops in your diffuser with some water and plug in. Let the aroma fill the air and breathe in the wellness and healing.

If you would like to apply directly to your skin, make sure you mix with a carrier oil such as fractionated coconut oil, or sweet almond oil. Mix 3 drops essentials with 6 drops carrier oil, and spread across your forehead.

Mix 1 drop per eight ounces tea for a warming healing drink... only use internally with great caution!

Another great way to indulge in these oils is with 10 drops or so in your bath water. Soak up the bliss and enjoy!

The Magic Blend

What you will need:

10 drops peppermint essential oil

10 drops lavender essential oil

5 drops grapefruit essential oil

5 drops valor essential oil

Directions:

Place 8-12 drops in your diffuser with some water and plug in. Let the aroma fill the air and breathe in the wellness and healing.

If you would like to apply directly to your skin, make sure you mix with a carrier oil such as fractionated coconut oil, or sweet almond oil. Mix 3 drops essentials with 6 drops carrier oil, and spread across your forehead.

Mix 1 drop per eight ounces tea for a warming healing drink... only use internally with great caution!

Another great way to indulge in these oils is with 10 drops or so in your bath water. Soak up the bliss and enjoy!

Your Best Friend Blend

What you will need:

10 drops frankincense essential oil

12 drops valor essential oil

10 drops thieves essential oil

4 drops myrrh oil

Directions:

Place 8-12 drops in your diffuser with some water and plug in. Let the aroma fill the air and breathe in the wellness and healing.

If you would like to apply directly to your skin, make sure you mix with a carrier oil such as fractionated coconut oil, or sweet almond oil. Mix 3 drops essentials with 6 drops carrier oil, and spread across your forehead.

Mix 1 drop per eight ounces tea for a warming healing drink... only use internally with great caution!

Another great way to indulge in these oils is with 10 drops or so in your bath water. Soak up the bliss and enjoy!

Conclusion

There you have it, everything you need to get started on your own essential oil journey. I know when you are first starting it can feel overwhelming, especially when you see the hundreds upon hundreds of essential oil options there are for you to choose from.

But, with this book, you are going to get the start you need to grow a collection, and learn how to use the oils you have for your greatest benefit. Take what you see here, and use it as inspiration for other blends, or simple find your favorites and stick with those.

There's no way you can go wrong when you are using essential oils, and with the inspiration in this book, you have what you need to make anything happen!

FREE Bonus Reminder

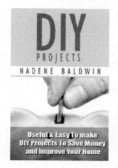

If you have not grabbed it yet, please go ahead and download your special bonus report *"DIY Projects. 13 Useful & Easy To Make DIY Projects To Save Money & Improve Your Home!"*

Simply Click the Button Below

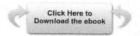

OR **Go to This Page**

http://diyhomecraft.com/free

BONUS #2: More Free & Discounted Books or Products

Do you want to receive more Free/Discounted Books or Products?

We have a mailing list where we send out our new Books or Products when they go free or with a discount on Amazon. Click on the link below to sign up for Free & Discount Book & Product Promotions.

=> Sign Up for Free & Discount Book & Product Promotions <=

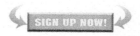

OR Go to this URL

http://zbit.ly/1WBb1Ek

Lightning Source UK Ltd.
Milton Keynes UK
UKOW05f2015050417

298451UK00006B/241/P